KEVIN HALL

Master Your Chronic Pain: With Nutrition and Targeted Treatments and Without Narcotics

Contents

1

Chapter 1: Understanding Chronic Pain

The first thing for you to know about chronic pain is that you are not alone. The second thing you need to know is that there are many effective remedies within your grasp that can take away or greatly reduce your pain. However, there is no "silver bullet" and to master your chronic pain you will have to approach it with patience and the willingness to try different remedies to determine a "best fit". But the first step towards mastery is understanding.

Chronic pain is a significant health issue worldwide, affecting millions of people. Its prevalence varies across different populations, but it's generally high, particularly among older adults. Estimates suggest that around 20% of adults globally suffer from chronic pain, with higher rates among certain people such as the elderly and individuals with certain medical conditions like arthritis or fibromyalgia. Inflammation lies at the heart of most chronic pain and the remedy is to reduce that inflammation.

The impact of chronic pain extends beyond physical discomfort and can profoundly affect individuals' quality of life. Some of the impacts include:

1. Physical Limitations: Chronic pain can restrict mobility and interfere with daily activities such as walking, standing, or even sitting for extended periods.
2. Emotional and Psychological Effects: Living with chronic pain can lead to depression, anxiety, and stress. It can also affect sleep patterns, leading to fatigue and exacerbating emotional distress.
3. Social Isolation: People experiencing chronic pain may withdraw from social activities due to discomfort or limitations, leading to feelings of isolation and loneliness.
4. Work and Financial Consequences: Chronic pain often leads to decreased productivity at work or even an inability to work altogether. This can result in financial strain due to medical expenses and loss of income.
5. Impact on Relationships: Chronic pain can strain relationships with family, friends, and caregivers due to the individual's limitations and emotional distress.

6. Increased Healthcare Utilization: Individuals with chronic pain often require frequent medical appointments, treatments, and medications, contributing to healthcare costs and potentially leading to dependency on pain management interventions.

So how does it work? What is the grip that chronic pain has on us?

Physical and psychological factors of chronic pain

Chronic pain is a complex phenomenon involving various physical and psychological mechanisms. Here are some key aspects of both:

1. Physical Mechanisms:

a. Peripheral Sensitization: In cases of injury or inflammation, peripheral nerves can become sensitized, leading to heightened sensitivity to pain stimuli. This can result in increased pain perception even in response to non-painful stimuli.

b. Central Sensitization: Chronic pain can involve changes in the central nervous system, particularly in the spinal cord and brain, leading to increased excitability of neurons. This amplifies pain signals and can result in persistent pain even after the initial injury or condition has healed.

c. Neurotransmitter Imbalance: Imbalances in neurotransmitters, such as serotonin, norepinephrine, and dopamine, can influence pain perception. For example, decreased levels of endogenous opioids (the body's natural painkillers) or increased levels of glutamate (an excitatory neurotransmitter) can contribute to chronic pain.

d. Structural Changes: Chronic pain conditions, such as arthritis or neuropathy, can cause structural changes in the affected tissues or nerves, leading to ongoing pain signals.

2. Psychological Mechanisms:

a. Cognitive Factors: Cognitive processes, such as attention, interpretation, and appraisal of pain signals, play a significant role in the experience of chronic pain. Negative thoughts, catastrophizing, and rumination can exacerbate pain perception and contribute to the development of chronic pain syndromes.

b. Emotional Factors: Emotional states, including stress, anxiety, and depression, can modulate pain perception through complex interactions with neurotransmitter systems and stress hormones. These emotional factors can also influence coping mechanisms and pain behaviors.

c. Social Factors: Social support, socioeconomic status, and cultural factors can impact how individuals experience and cope with chronic pain. Lack of support or stigmatization can exacerbate feelings of isolation and distress, further amplifying pain perception.

d. Behavioral Factors: Pain-related behaviors, such as avoidance of activities or overreliance on medication, can perpetuate the cycle of chronic pain. Maladaptive coping strategies, such as substance abuse or withdrawal from social interactions, can also contribute to the maintenance of chronic pain conditions.

Understanding the interplay between these physical and psychological mechanisms is crucial for you and your provider developing a comprehensive treatment approach for managing your pain. Effective interventions often involve a combination of pharmacological treatments, physical therapies, psychological interventions (such as cognitive-behavioral therapy), and lifestyle modifications tailored to address both the physical and psychological aspects of chronic pain.

2

Chapter 2: The Role of Nutrition in Chronic Pain

The relationship between diet and chronic pain is a complex and multifaceted one, with various factors contributing to how diet influences pain perception and management. While diet alone may not be a cure for chronic pain conditions, it can play a significant role in either exacerbating or alleviating symptoms. Here are some key points to consider regarding the relationship between diet and chronic pain:

1. Inflammation: Chronic pain is often associated with inflammation in the body. Certain foods can either promote or reduce inflammation. Foods high in refined sugars, saturated fats, and processed ingredients can contribute to inflammation, worsening pain symptoms. On the other hand, a diet rich in fruits, vegetables, whole grains, healthy fats (such as those found in nuts, seeds, and fatty fish), and antioxidants can help reduce inflammation and potentially alleviate pain.

2. Weight Management: Carrying excess weight can put added stress on joints and exacerbate pain in conditions such as osteoarthritis. A balanced diet that supports weight management can help reduce strain on the body and alleviate pain symptoms associated with carrying excess weight.

3. Nutrient Deficiencies: Certain nutrients play crucial roles in pain modulation and overall bodily function. For example, deficiencies in vitamins D and B12 have been linked to increased pain sensitivity. Ensuring adequate intake of essential nutrients through a balanced diet or supplementation may help manage chronic pain conditions.

4. Gut Health: Emerging research suggests a link between gut health and chronic pain. The gut microbiota, influenced by diet, can affect systemic inflammation and pain perception. Diets high in fiber and probiotics (found in fermented foods like yogurt and kefir) can support a healthy gut microbiome, potentially reducing inflammation and improving pain symptoms.

5. Food Sensitivities: Some individuals may have food sensitivities or intolerances that can exacerbate chronic pain symptoms. Common culprits include gluten, dairy, and certain artificial additives. Identifying and eliminating trigger foods from the diet may help reduce inflammation and alleviate pain in susceptible individuals.

6. Hydration: Dehydration can exacerbate pain symptoms, particularly headaches and joint pain. Maintaining proper hydration by drinking an adequate amount of water throughout the day can help manage chronic pain.

7. Psychological Factors: Diet can also influence mood and mental health, which in turn can impact pain perception.

Consuming a diet rich in whole foods and nutrients that support brain health, such as omega-3 fatty acids, can help maintain emotional well-being and potentially reduce the impact of psychological factors on chronic pain.

It's important to note that individual responses to dietary changes can vary, and what works for one person may not work for another. Finding a provider who will work with you to integrate dietary changes with other pain management strategies, such as physical therapy, medication, and stress management techniques, offer comprehensive support for individuals living with chronic pain.

Here are some examples of foods that may exacerbate or ease chronic pain:

Foods that may exacerbate chronic pain:

1. Processed Foods: Foods high in refined sugars, unhealthy fats, and artificial additives can contribute to inflammation and exacerbate pain symptoms. Examples include fast food, sugary snacks, and processed meats.
2. Saturated Fats: Foods high in saturated fats, such as red meat, full-fat dairy products, and fried foods, can promote inflammation and worsen chronic pain conditions.
3. Trans Fats: Trans fats, found in partially hydrogenated oils often used in processed and fried foods, have been linked to increased inflammation and may exacerbate pain symptoms.
4. Refined Carbohydrates: Foods made with refined grains, such as white bread, white rice, and pastries, can cause spikes in blood sugar levels and contribute to inflammation, potentially worsening chronic pain.

5. Alcohol: Excessive alcohol consumption can disrupt sleep patterns, increase inflammation, and interfere with the body's ability to manage pain, making chronic pain symptoms more pronounced.

6. High-Sodium Foods: A diet high in sodium can lead to water retention and exacerbate inflammation, potentially worsening pain symptoms. Processed foods, canned soups, and fast food are common sources of excessive sodium.

7. Nightshade Vegetables: Some individuals with chronic pain conditions, particularly arthritis, report sensitivity to nightshade vegetables such as tomatoes, peppers, eggplants, and potatoes. These vegetables contain alkaloids that may contribute to inflammation and pain in susceptible individuals.

Foods that may ease chronic pain:

1. Fruits and Vegetables: Colorful fruits and vegetables are rich in antioxidants and anti-inflammatory compounds, which can help reduce inflammation and alleviate pain. Examples include berries, leafy greens, broccoli, and bell peppers.

2. Fatty Fish: Cold-water fatty fish such as salmon, mackerel, and sardines are rich in omega-3 fatty acids, which have anti-inflammatory properties and may help alleviate chronic pain symptoms.

3. Nuts and Seeds: Nuts and seeds, such as walnuts, almonds, flaxseeds, and chia seeds, are excellent sources of healthy fats and antioxidants, which can help reduce inflammation

and support overall health.

4. Whole Grains: Whole grains like oats, quinoa, brown rice, and whole wheat are rich in fiber and nutrients that can help stabilize blood sugar levels and reduce inflammation, potentially easing chronic pain.

5. Herbs and Spices: Certain herbs and spices have anti-inflammatory properties and may help alleviate pain. Examples include turmeric, ginger, cinnamon, and garlic.

6. Healthy Oils: Olive oil, avocado oil, and coconut oil are rich in monounsaturated fats and antioxidants, which can help reduce inflammation and support overall health.

7. Protein Sources: Lean sources of protein such as poultry, tofu, beans, and lentils provide essential nutrients that support muscle health and may help alleviate pain associated with conditions like fibromyalgia.

8. Vitamin D: Adequate vitamin D levels are important for bone health and immune function. Some research suggests that vitamin D deficiency may be associated with increased pain sensitivity and chronic pain conditions. Foods rich in vitamin D include fatty fish, fortified dairy products, and egg yolks. Sunlight exposure is also a natural source of vitamin D.

9. Magnesium: Magnesium plays a role in muscle relaxation and nerve function. Low magnesium levels have been linked to increased pain sensitivity and muscle cramps. Foods high in magnesium include leafy green vegetables, nuts, seeds, whole grains, and legumes.

10. Vitamin B12: Vitamin B12 is important for nerve health and function. Deficiency in vitamin B12 can lead to neuropathic pain and other neurological symptoms. Food sources of vitamin B12

include meat, fish, eggs, dairy products, and fortified cereals.

11. Turmeric/Curcumin: Curcumin, the active compound in turmeric, has potent anti-inflammatory and antioxidant properties. It may help alleviate pain and inflammation in conditions such as arthritis. Turmeric can be incorporated into cooking or consumed as a supplement. Remember to add black pepper to turmeric, this greatly enhances the anti-inflammatory potency.

12. Ginger: Ginger has anti-inflammatory properties and may help reduce pain and inflammation associated with conditions such as osteoarthritis and muscle soreness. It can be consumed fresh, dried, or as a supplement.

13. Glucosamine and Chondroitin: These are natural compounds found in cartilage. They are often taken as supplements to support joint health and may help reduce pain and improve mobility in individuals with osteoarthritis.

14. Essential Amino Acids: Amino acids are the building blocks of proteins, which are essential for tissue repair and muscle function. Consuming adequate amounts of high-quality protein sources, such as lean meats, poultry, fish, eggs, dairy products, and plant-based proteins, can support overall health and aid in pain management.

Choosing what you eat is very important in bringing you long-term results that will benefit you for a lifetime, not just for chronic pain but in many aspects of your overall health. Nutrition can be a powerful ally in controlling your inflammation, and inflammation is at the heart of a great many chronic conditions.

3

Chapter 3: Targeted Therapies

Non-drug solutions for chronic pain management encompass a wide range of interventions that aim to alleviate pain, improve function, and enhance overall well-being without relying on pharmaceutical medications. Here are some common non-drug approaches, along with how they work and their effectiveness:

1. Physical Therapy:

- How it works: Physical therapy involves exercises, stretches, manual therapy techniques, and modalities such as heat, cold, or electrical stimulation to improve strength, flexibility, and mobility, as well as to reduce pain and inflammation.

- Effectiveness: Physical therapy is often highly effective for chronic pain, particularly musculoskeletal conditions like low back pain, osteoarthritis, and fibromyalgia. Research has shown that structured exercise programs and manual therapy can lead to significant improvements in pain and function.

2. Exercise:

- How it works: Regular physical activity can help strengthen muscles, improve joint flexibility, release endorphins (natural painkillers), and reduce inflammation, leading to decreased pain perception and improved overall health.

- Effectiveness: Exercise has been shown to be beneficial for various chronic pain conditions, including arthritis, chronic low back pain, and fibromyalgia. Both aerobic exercises (e.g., walking, swimming) and strength training can contribute to pain relief and improved function.

3. Cognitive-Behavioral Therapy (CBT):

- How it works: CBT focuses on identifying and changing negative thoughts, beliefs, and behaviors associated with pain. It teaches coping skills, relaxation techniques, and stress management strategies to help individuals better manage their pain and improve their quality of life.

- Effectiveness: CBT has been found to be effective in reducing pain intensity, improving mood, and enhancing coping abilities in individuals with chronic pain. It can also lead to long-lasting improvements in pain-related outcomes.

4. Mindfulness Meditation:

- How it works: Mindfulness meditation involves cultivating awareness of the present moment without judgment. By practicing mindfulness techniques, individuals learn to observe their pain sensations without becoming overwhelmed by them, which can lead to decreased pain perception and improved emotional well-being.

- Effectiveness: Research suggests that mindfulness meditation can be effective in reducing pain severity, increasing pain tolerance, and improving psychological outcomes such as depression and anxiety in individuals with chronic pain.

5. Acupuncture:

- How it works: Acupuncture involves the insertion of thin needles into specific points on the body to stimulate nerves, muscles, and connective tissues. This stimulation is thought to modulate pain signals, promote the release of endorphins, and restore the body's natural balance.

- Effectiveness: While the evidence for acupuncture's effectiveness in chronic pain management is mixed, some studies suggest that it may provide relief for conditions such as osteoarthritis, migraines, and chronic low back pain. Individual responses to acupuncture can vary, and it may be more effective for some individuals than others.

6. Biofeedback:

- How it works: Biofeedback involves using electronic monitoring devices to provide real-time feedback on physiological processes such as muscle tension, heart rate, and skin temperature. By learning to control these bodily functions, individuals can reduce stress levels and alleviate pain.

- Effectiveness: Biofeedback has been shown to be effective in reducing pain intensity, improving physical function, and enhancing overall quality of life in individuals with chronic pain, particularly tension-type headaches, migraines, and temporomandibular joint disorder (TMJ).

These non-drug solutions for chronic pain management are often most effective when used as part of a comprehensive treatment plan tailored to your specific needs and preferences. Integrating multiple approaches, such as combining physical therapy with cognitive-behavioral therapy or mindfulness meditation, can maximize the benefits and improve outcomes for individuals living with chronic pain.

4

Chapter 4: Holistic Approaches for Pain Management

The mind-body connection is where holistic approaches lead us. The mind-body connection plays a crucial role in treating chronic pain as it involves the interplay between psychological and physiological factors. By understanding and harnessing this connection, individuals can potentially reduce pain perception, improve coping mechanisms, and enhance overall well-being. Here's an explanation of the mind-body connection in treating chronic pain and approaches to increase it:

1. Psychological Techniques:

- Cognitive-Behavioral Therapy (CBT): CBT aims to change negative thought patterns and behaviors that contribute to pain perception. By identifying and challenging maladaptive beliefs about pain, individuals can develop healthier coping strategies and reduce distress.

- Mindfulness-Based Stress Reduction (MBSR): MBSR teaches mindfulness meditation techniques to increase awareness of the present moment without judgment. Practicing mindfulness can help individuals observe pain sensations without reacting to them emotionally, thereby reducing suffering.

- Relaxation Techniques: Techniques such as progressive muscle relaxation, deep breathing exercises, and guided imagery can help reduce muscle tension, alleviate stress, and promote relaxation, which may indirectly reduce pain intensity.

- Biofeedback: Biofeedback involves using electronic monitoring devices to provide real-time feedback about physiological processes such as muscle tension or skin temperature. By learning to control these bodily functions, individuals can gain a sense of mastery over their symptoms and reduce pain perception.

2. Physical Techniques:

- Yoga and Tai Chi: These mind-body practices combine physical postures, breathing exercises, and meditation to promote relaxation, flexibility, and balance. Regular practice of yoga or Tai Chi may help reduce pain intensity, improve functional mobility, and enhance overall well-being.

- Acupuncture: Acupuncture involves the insertion of thin needles into specific points on the body to stimulate nerve pathways and release endorphins, the body's natural painkillers. Acupuncture may help alleviate chronic pain by modulating pain signals and promoting relaxation.

- Massage Therapy: Massage therapy can help reduce muscle tension, improve blood circulation, and promote relaxation, which may provide temporary relief from chronic pain. Different massage techniques, such as Swedish massage or deep tissue massage, may be beneficial depending on the individual's preferences and pain condition.

3. Educational and Self-Management Approaches:

- Pain Education: Understanding the biopsychosocial factors

contributing to chronic pain can empower individuals to take an active role in managing their symptoms. Education about pain physiology, lifestyle modifications, and self-care strategies can help individuals make informed decisions about their health. This book is a great first step.

- Self-Management Programs: Participating in self-management programs, such as pain management workshops or peer support groups, can provide practical tools and emotional support for coping with chronic pain. Peer support can reduce feelings of isolation and provide validation for shared experiences.

Increasing the mind-body connection involves cultivating awareness of the interactions between thoughts, emotions, sensations, and behaviors. This can be achieved through regular practice of mindfulness, relaxation techniques, and other mind-body interventions. Developing a holistic approach to pain management that addresses both the physical and psychological aspects of pain is key to improving outcomes and enhancing overall quality of life for individuals living with chronic pain.Somethings are mentioned several times in this book, it is effort to provide linkage between certain solutions.

Chapter 5: Alternative Treatments for Chronic Pain

In addition to the mind-body techniques mentioned earlier, there are several alternative treatments for chronic pain that individuals may consider. While these approaches may offer benefits for some people, it's essential to recognize that their effectiveness can vary, and they may not be suitable for everyone. Here are some alternative treatments for chronic pain, along with their benefits and limitations:

1.Chiropractic Care:

- Benefits: Chiropractic care involves manual manipulation of the spine and musculoskeletal system to improve alignment and reduce pain. It may be beneficial for certain types of musculoskeletal pain, such as back pain and neck pain. Chiropractic adjustments can help alleviate joint stiffness, improve mobility, and promote overall well-being.

- Limitations: While chiropractic care is generally considered safe when performed by a qualified practitioner, it may not be appropriate for all types of chronic pain or underlying medical conditions. Some individuals may experience temporary soreness or discomfort after treatment. Additionally, the evidence supporting the effectiveness of chiropractic care for chronic pain is mixed, and more research is needed to determine its long-term benefits.

2. Acupuncture:

- Benefits: Acupuncture involves the insertion of thin needles into specific points on the body to stimulate nerve pathways and promote healing. It may help alleviate chronic pain by modulating pain signals, reducing inflammation, and promoting relaxation. Acupuncture is generally well-tolerated and may provide relief for conditions such as osteoarthritis, fibromyalgia, and headache disorders.

- Limitations: While acupuncture is considered safe when performed by a trained practitioner using sterile needles, it may not be suitable for individuals with certain medical conditions or those who are unwilling to try needle-based therapies. The evidence supporting the effectiveness of acupuncture for chronic pain is mixed, and individual responses can vary.

3. Herbal Remedies and Supplements:

- Benefits: Some herbal remedies and dietary supplements, such as turmeric, ginger, and omega-3 fatty acids, have anti-inflammatory properties and may help reduce pain and inflammation associated with chronic conditions such as arthritis. Additionally, certain supplements, such as glucosamine and chondroitin, may support joint health and improve mobility.

- Limitations: Herbal remedies and supplements are not regulated as rigorously as pharmaceutical drugs, and their safety and efficacy may vary. It's essential to consult with a healthcare provider before taking any herbal remedies or supplements, especially if you have underlying health conditions or are taking medications, as they may interact with other treatments.

4. Transcutaneous Electrical Nerve Stimulation (TENS):

- Benefits: TENS therapy involves the use of low-voltage electrical currents to stimulate nerve fibers and reduce pain perception. It may help alleviate chronic pain by blocking pain signals and promoting the release of endorphins, the body's natural painkillers. TENS therapy is non-invasive, portable, and can be used at home.

- Limitations: While TENS therapy is generally safe and well-tolerated, its effectiveness for chronic pain can vary, and some individuals may not experience significant relief. TENS may not be suitable for certain types of pain or underlying medical conditions, and it's essential to use the device properly to avoid adverse effects.

5. Meditation and Relaxation Techniques:

- Benefits: Meditation, mindfulness, and relaxation techniques such as deep breathing exercises and progressive muscle relaxation can help reduce stress, alleviate muscle tension, and promote a sense of calmness. These practices may indirectly reduce pain intensity and improve overall well-being in individuals with chronic pain conditions.

- Limitations: While meditation and relaxation techniques are generally safe and accessible, they may require consistent practice and may not provide immediate relief for severe pain episodes. Additionally, some individuals may find it challenging to maintain focus or achieve relaxation, especially in the presence of ongoing pain.

6. Physical Therapy:

- Benefits: Physical therapy involves exercises, manual techniques, and other modalities to improve strength, flexibility, and functional mobility. It may help individuals with chronic pain learn proper body mechanics, reduce muscle imbalances, and improve posture, which can alleviate pain and prevent further injury.

-Limitations: While physical therapy can be highly effective for certain types of chronic pain, such as musculoskeletal conditions, it may require a significant time commitment and consistency to achieve lasting results. Additionally, access to physical therapy services may be limited, particularly in underserved areas or for individuals with financial constraints.

7. PEMF (Pulsed Electromagnetic Field) therapy is a non-invasive treatment modality that has been explored for its potential benefits in managing chronic pain.

Benefits: PEMF therapy has shown promise in providing relief from chronic pain conditions such as osteoarthritis, fibromyalgia, and neuropathic pain. The electromagnetic fields generated by PEMF devices may help modulate pain signals and reduce pain perception. PEMF therapy has been found to possess anti-inflammatory properties, which can be beneficial for individuals suffering from chronic pain associated with inflammation. By reducing inflammation, PEMF therapy may help alleviate pain symptoms and improve overall function. PEMF therapy has been shown to stimulate tissue repair and regeneration processes. It may promote the healing of musculoskeletal injuries, such as fractures and soft tissue injuries, which can contribute to chronic pain if left untreated. PEMF therapy is non-invasive and generally considered safe when used appropriately. Unlike invasive procedures or pharmaceutical interventions, PEMF therapy typically involves minimal risk of adverse effects when administered by a trained professional. PEMF therapy can often be administered in clinical settings or at home using portable devices. This convenience allows individuals to incorporate

PEMF therapy into their pain management regimen without significant disruption to their daily routine.

Limitations: While there is some evidence supporting the efficacy of PEMF therapy for chronic pain management, the research in this area is still relatively limited. More high-quality studies are needed to fully understand the effectiveness of PEMF therapy across different types of chronic pain conditions and patient populations. Responses to PEMF therapy can vary widely among individuals. Factors such as the specific condition being treated, the severity of symptoms, and individual differences in physiology may influence the effectiveness of PEMF therapy for pain relief. The cost of PEMF therapy devices can vary depending on factors such as the type of device, its features, and whether it is intended for clinical or home use. While some individuals may find PEMF therapy cost-effective in the long run, others may find it financially prohibitive, especially if insurance coverage is limited. Achieving optimal results with PEMF therapy may require regular and consistent use over an extended period. Individuals may need to commit to multiple sessions per week or daily treatments to experience significant pain relief and other therapeutic benefits. PEMF therapy may not be suitable for individuals with certain medical conditions or implanted medical devices, such as pacemakers or cochlear implants. It's essential for individuals to consult with a healthcare professional before initiating PEMF therapy to ensure its safety and appropriateness for their specific situation.

It's essential to approach alternative treatments for chronic pain with caution and to consult with a healthcare provider and trained practitioners, before trying any new therapy, especially if you have underlying medical conditions or are taking medications. Integrating alternative treatments into a comprehensive pain management plan that includes conventional medical interventions, lifestyle modifications, and psychological support can help optimize outcomes and improve quality of life for individuals living with chronic pain.

6

Chapter 6: Lifestyle adjustment for Pain Relief

A change in lifestyle is often a large concern of people with chronic pain. Lifestyle considerations such as sleep, exercise, and stress management play a crucial role in mastering chronic pain. These factors can significantly influence pain perception, physical function, and overall well-being. Here's an explanation of their importance and some practical tips for improving sleep quality and quantity, exercise, and stress management in individuals with chronic pain:

Sleep: **Importance**: Quality sleep is essential for tissue repair, immune function, and overall health. Poor sleep can exacerbate pain sensitivity, increase inflammation, and impair cognitive function, making it harder to cope with chronic pain.

Tips for Improving Sleep:

Maintain a Consistent Sleep Schedule: Go to bed and wake up at the same time every day, even on weekends, to regulate your body's internal clock.

Create a Relaxing Bedtime Routine: Establish calming activities before bed, such as reading, taking a warm bath, or practicing relaxation techniques like deep breathing or meditation.

Create a Comfortable Sleep Environment: Make sure your bedroom is conducive to sleep by keeping it dark, quiet, and cool. Invest in a comfortable mattress and pillows that support your body.

Limit Stimulants and Screen Time: Avoid caffeine, nicotine, and electronics (e.g., smartphones, computers, TVs) at least an hour before bedtime, as they can interfere with sleep quality.

Manage Pain Before Bed: Use pain management techniques such as heat therapy, gentle stretching, or over-the-counter pain relievers as needed to alleviate discomfort before bedtime.

Exercise:

Importance: Regular physical activity can improve muscle strength, flexibility, and cardiovascular health. Exercise also releases endorphins, which are natural pain relievers, and promotes better sleep and mood regulation.

Tips for Incorporating Exercise:

Start Slowly and Gradually Increase Intensity: Begin with low-impact activities such as walking, swimming, or cycling, and gradually increase duration and intensity as tolerated.

Choose Activities You Enjoy: Find enjoyable activities that fit your interests and physical abilities, whether it's yoga, gardening, dancing, or tai chi. Variety can help prevent boredom and maintain motivation.

Focus on Consistency: Aim for at least 150 minutes of moderate-intensity aerobic exercise per week, spread throughout the week.

Incorporate strength training exercises at least twice a week to improve muscle strength and function.

Listen to Your Body: Pay attention to your body's signals and adjust your exercise routine accordingly. Rest when needed and avoid pushing through pain that exacerbates your symptoms.

Stress Management:

Importance: Chronic pain and stress have a bidirectional relationship, with stress exacerbating pain and pain increasing stress levels. Effective stress management techniques can help break this cycle and improve overall well-being.

Tips for Managing Stress:

Practice Relaxation Techniques: Incorporate relaxation techniques such as deep breathing exercises, progressive muscle relaxation, guided imagery, or mindfulness meditation into your daily routine.

Engage in Enjoyable Activities: Make time for activities that bring you joy and relaxation, whether it's spending time in nature, listening to music, practicing hobbies, or spending time with loved ones.

Set Realistic Expectations: Prioritize tasks and delegate responsibilities to avoid feeling overwhelmed. Break tasks into smaller, manageable steps and celebrate your accomplishments.

Seek Support: Talk to friends, family members, or a mental

health professional about your feelings and concerns. Joining support groups or attending counseling sessions can provide validation, guidance, and coping strategies for managing stress.

By prioritizing sleep, exercise, and stress management, individuals with chronic pain will enhance their overall quality of life, improve pain management, and cultivate resilience in the face of challenges. It's essential to experiment with different strategies and tailor them to your individual needs and preferences to find what works best for you. Additionally, consulting with healthcare professionals, such as physical therapists, pain specialists, or psychologists, can provide personalized guidance and support in implementing lifestyle changes for chronic pain management.

7

Chapter 7: The Importance of Social Support in Pain Management

Social support and social connections can play a significant role in chronic pain management by providing emotional encouragement, practical assistance, and a sense of belonging. Here's how social support can benefit individuals with chronic pain and some ways to find and grow social support:

Emotional Support:

Validation and Understanding: Having someone who listens empathetically and validates your experiences can help reduce feelings of isolation and distress associated with chronic pain.

Encouragement and Motivation: Supportive friends, family members, or peers can provide encouragement and motivation to engage in pain management strategies, such as exercise, relaxation techniques, or seeking professional help.

1. **Practical Support**:

· **Assistance with Daily Tasks**: Friends or family members can offer practical assistance with daily tasks, such as household chores, errands, or transportation, especially during times when pain levels are high or mobility is limited.

- **Accompaniment to Appointments**: Having someone accompany you to medical appointments or therapy sessions can provide emotional support and help ensure that important information is communicated and understood.

2.) Sense of Belonging and Connection:

- **Reduced Feelings of Isolation**: Social connections can reduce feelings of loneliness and isolation commonly experienced by individuals with chronic pain. Engaging in meaningful social interactions can foster a sense of belonging and connectedness.
- **Shared Experiences**: Connecting with others who have similar experiences with chronic pain can provide validation, empathy, and shared coping strategies. Peer support groups or online communities can be valuable resources for finding solidarity and understanding.

1. **Distraction and Enjoyment**:

- **Engaging in Social Activities**: Participating in social activities, hobbies, or leisure pursuits with friends or family members can provide enjoyable distractions from pain and promote positive emotions.

Ways to Find and Grow Social Support:

1. **Cultivate Existing Relationships**:

- **Communicate Openly**: Share your experiences, needs, and feelings with trusted friends, family members, or colleagues. Open communication can strengthen relationships and foster understanding.
- **Express Gratitude**: Show appreciation for the support you receive from others, whether through verbal acknowledgment, gestures of kindness, or reciprocal acts of support.

1. **Seek Out Supportive Communities**:

- **Join Support Groups**: Look for local or online support groups specifically for individuals living with chronic pain. These groups offer opportunities to connect with others, share experiences, and exchange coping strategies.
- **Attend Educational Workshops**: Participate in workshops or seminars focused on chronic pain management, where you can meet others facing similar challenges and learn from experts in the field.

1. **Explore Peer Mentoring Programs**:

- **Peer Support Programs**: Consider participating in peer mentoring programs where individuals with lived experiences of chronic pain provide guidance, encouragement, and practical advice to others who are newly diagnosed or struggling to manage their symptoms.

1. **Utilize Technology**:

- **Online Communities and Forums**: Explore online forums, social media groups, or virtual support communities dedicated to chronic pain management. These platforms offer opportunities for anonymous sharing, networking, and support from individuals worldwide.

1. **Engage in Social Activities**:

- **Attend Social Events**: Participate in social events, gatherings, or recreational activities that align with your interests and abilities. Join clubs, classes, or community organizations where you can meet new people and build connections over shared hobbies or passions.

By actively seeking out social support and nurturing existing relationships, individuals with chronic pain can build a strong support network that enhances their resilience, coping skills, and overall well-being. Remember that it's beneficial to ask for help and that seeking support is a sign of strength, not weakness.

8

Chapter 8: Building Resilience in the Face of Chronic Pain

Cognitive reframing and gratitude practice are psychological techniques that build resilience and play a crucial role in preventing relapse and maintaining long-term success in managing chronic pain:

1. Cognitive Reframing:
   - Importance: Cognitive reframing involves shifting one's perspective or interpretation of a situation to create a more positive or adaptive outlook. In the context of chronic pain, cognitive reframing can help individuals reinterpret pain sensations, reduce catastrophic thinking, and develop more adaptive coping strategies.
   - Benefits: By reframing negative thoughts and beliefs about pain, individuals can reduce emotional distress, improve pain tolerance, and enhance overall well-being. Cognitive reframing can also empower individuals to regain a sense of control over

their lives and focus on achievable goals.

- Strategies: Cognitive-behavioral therapy (CBT) techniques, such as cognitive restructuring and thought challenging, can be effective for teaching individuals how to identify and reframe unhelpful thoughts related to pain. Practicing mindfulness meditation and acceptance-based approaches, such as Acceptance and Commitment Therapy (ACT), can also promote cognitive flexibility and acceptance of pain-related experiences.

2. Gratitude Practice:

- Importance: Gratitude practice involves intentionally cultivating appreciation and thankfulness for positive aspects of one's life, despite the presence of challenges or difficulties such as chronic pain. Gratitude practice can help individuals shift their focus away from pain and towards experiences of joy, connection, and resilience.

- Benefits: Regular gratitude practice has been associated with improved mood, reduced stress, and enhanced resilience in the face of adversity. By fostering a sense of gratitude, individuals can develop a more positive outlook on life, strengthen social relationships, and increase their overall sense of well-being.

- Strategies: Keep a gratitude journal and write down three things you're grateful for each day, focusing on simple pleasures, acts of kindness, or moments of connection. Practice expressing gratitude verbally or through written notes to loved ones, caregivers, or healthcare providers. Incorporate gratitude rituals into daily routines, such as saying a thank-you prayer before meals or reflecting on moments of gratitude before bedtime

9

Chapter 9: Strategies for Maintaining Long-Term Success and Freedom from Chronic Pain

1. Consistent Pain Management Practices: Continue with evidence-based pain management strategies that have been effective in reducing pain and improving function, such as medication management, physical therapy, and psychological interventions.

2. Healthy Lifestyle Habits: Maintain a healthy lifestyle by prioritizing regular exercise, balanced nutrition, adequate sleep, and stress management techniques. These lifestyle factors can contribute to overall well-being and resilience against pain.

3. Regular Monitoring and Self-Care: Stay vigilant about monitoring pain symptoms and addressing any changes or flare-ups promptly. Practice self-care activities that promote

relaxation, such as meditation, deep breathing exercises, or engaging in hobbies and interests.

4. Social Support and Connection: Cultivate supportive relationships with friends, family members, support groups, or healthcare professionals who understand and validate your experiences with chronic pain. Lean on your support network during challenging times and share your successes and achievements with others.

5. Flexibility and Adaptability: Be flexible and adaptable in your approach to pain management, recognizing that strategies that worked in the past may need to be adjusted over time. Stay open to trying new techniques or therapies that may offer additional relief or support.

6. Positive Mindset and Resilience: Cultivate a positive mindset and resilience by focusing on strengths, cultivating gratitude, and embracing moments of joy and connection in your life. Practice self-compassion and acknowledge your efforts and progress in managing chronic pain.

By incorporating cognitive reframing, gratitude practice, and other evidence-based strategies into a comprehensive pain management plan, you can reduce the risk of relapse and maintain long-term success and freedom from the debilitating effects of persistent pain. It's essential to work closely with healthcare providers to tailor treatment approaches to individual needs and goals and to seek support from a multidisciplinary team when needed. Remember, where we first began, you are not alone in conquering chronic pain.

If this book has helped you please write a favorable review at Amazon

10

Resources

- Addressing chronic pain requires a comprehensive approach that may include medical treatments, physical therapy, psychological support, lifestyle modifications, and social support networks. It's essential to recognize the multi-faceted impact of chronic pain and Cheng C-A, Chiu Y-W, Wu D, et al. Effectiveness of tai chi on fibromyalgia patients: a meta-analysis of randomized controlled trials. *Complementary Therapies in Medicine.* 2019;46:1-8.
- Chou R, Deyo R, Friedly J, et al. Nonpharmacologic therapies for low back pain: a systematic review for an American College of Physicians clinical practice guideline. *Annals of Internal Medicine.* 2017;166(7):493-505.
- Coulter ID, Crawford C, Vernon H, et al. Manipulation and mobilization for treating chronic nonspecific neck pain: a systematic review and meta-analysis for an appropriateness panel. *Pain Physician.* 2019;22(2):E55-E70.

- Dowell D, Ragan KR, Jones CM, et al. CDC clinical practice guideline for prescribing opioids for pain—United States, 2022. *MMWR. Morbidity and Mortality Weekly Report.* 2022;71(3):1-95.
- Furlan AD, Giraldo M, Baskwill A, et al. Massage for low-back pain. *Cochrane Database of Systematic Reviews.* 2015;(9):CD001929. Accessed at cochranelibrary.com on November 8, 2022.
- Garza-Villareal EA, Pando V, Vuust P, et al. Music-induced analgesia in chronic pain conditions: a systematic review and meta-analysis. *Pain Physician.* 2017;20(7):597-610.
- Institute of Medicine. *Relieving Pain in America: A Blueprint for Transforming Prevention, Care, Education, and Research.* The National Academies Press website. Accessed at nap.edu/catalog/13172/relieving-pain-in-america-a-blueprint-for-transforming-prevention-care on November 8, 2022.
- Kolasinski SL, Neogi T, Hochberg MC, et al. 2019 American College of Rheumatology/Arthritis Foundation guideline for the management of osteoarthritis of the hand, hip, and knee. *Arthritis & Rheumatology.* 2020;72(2):220-233.
- Lacy BE, Pimentel M, Brenner DM, et al. ACG clinical guideline: management of irritable bowel syndrome. *American Journal of Gastroenterology.* 2021;116(1):17-44.
- Lin Y-C, Wan L, Jamison RN. Using integrative medicine in pain management: an evaluation of current evidence. *Anesthesia and Analgesia.* 2017;125(6):2081-2093.
- Qaseem A, Wilt TJ, McLean RM, et al. Noninvasive treatments for acute, subacute, and chronic low back pain: a clinical practice guideline from the American College of Physicians. *Annals of Internal Medicine.* 2017;166(7):514-530.

- Rist PM, Hernandez A, Bernstein C, et al. The impact of spinal manipulation on migraine pain and disability: a systematic review and meta-analysis. *Headache.* 2019;59(4):532-542.
- Vickers AJ, Vertosick EA, Lewith G, et al. Acupuncture for chronic pain: update of an individual patient data meta-analysis. *Journal of Pain.* 2018;19(5):455-474.
- Non-Drug Pain Management: MedlinePlus